Vegetarian Grilling Cookbook

The Best Recipes for Grilling Delicious
Vegetarian Dishes on the Grill

By
Linda Parker

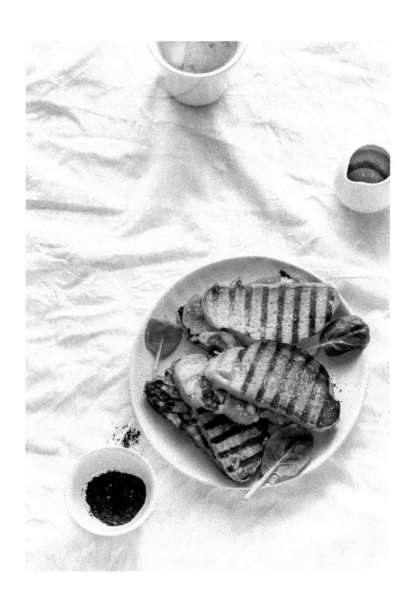

Table of Contents

Introduction

Vegetarianism refers to a lifestyle that excludes the consumption of all forms of meat including pork, chicken, beef, lamb, venison, fish, and shells. Depending on a person's belief and lifestyle, vegetarianism has different spectrums. There are vegetarians, who like to consume products that come from animals such as milk, eggs, cream and cheese. On the other end of that spectrum are the vegans. Vegans never consume meat or any product that comes from animals.

Benefits of Vegetarianism

According to research, living a vegetarian lifestyle lowers your risk of getting some of the major chronic diseases such as heart disease, cancer and type 2 diabetes. Vegetarians are 19 to 25% less likely to die of any kind of heart disease. The high consumption of fiber from grains also prevents the blood sugar spikes that lead to heart attacks and diabetes. The consumption of nuts, which are high in fiber, antioxidants and omega 3 fatty acids also helps lower the vegetarian's risk of getting heart attacks.

Due to the avoidance of red meat, you'll also eliminate a great deal of risk in getting certain types of cancer such as colon cancer. The high level of antioxidants from green leafy vegetables and fruits also helps in this area.

What About These Missing Nutrients?

Some people may be concerned with the lack of the following nutrients in a vegetarian diet however you'll find that there are certain types of vegetables and fruits that can supply these nutrients to give you a perfectly balanced diet. Some of the nutrients of concern are protein, iron, calcium and vitamin b12.

Protein can easily be found in beans and products made from beans such as tofu. Nuts and peas are also good sources of protein. Iron can also be found in tofu, beans, spinach, chard and cashews. Calcium can easily be found in soy milk, broccoli, collard greens, mustard greens and kale.

How to Make The Change

When you're starting out with this lifestyle, you might want to take baby steps. Start with 1 vegetarian meal per day. This allows you to adapt gradually to the different taste and flavors of a vegetarian diet. Once you're used to having a vegetarian meal every day, you can slowly add one more vegetarian meal until you've completely changed your lifestyle. Research has found that making small changes is more sustainable in the end. It's not a contest. Take your time and enjoy the different types of vegetarian meals. How To Use This Book As you browse through the pages, figure out which recipes you like and make them a part of your daily life. This book is filled with different types of vegan dishes and some of them include classic dishes that have been adapted to suit the vegan diet.

Grilled Zucchini and Cremini Mushrooms with Balsamic Glaze

Ingredients:

- 3 yellow bell peppers, seeded and halved
- 3 summer squash (about 1 pound total), sliced lengthwise into 1/2-inch-thick rectangles
- 3 zucchini (about 12 ounces total), sliced lengthwise into 1/2-inch-thick rectangles
- 3 eggplant (12 ounces total), sliced lengthwise into 1/2-inch-thick rectangles
- 12 cremini mushrooms
- 1 bunch (1-pound) asparagus, trimmed
- 12 green onions, roots cut off
- 6 tablespoons olive oil
- Salt and freshly ground black pepper
- 3 tablespoons balsamic vinegar
- 4 garlic cloves, minced
- 1 teaspoon chopped fresh parsley leaves
- 1 teaspoon chopped fresh basil leaves
- 1/2 teaspoon finely chopped fresh rosemary leaves

Directions:

1. Preheat your grill for medium-high heat.
2. Lightly brush the vegetables with 1/4 cup of the oil.
3. Season the vegetables with salt and pepper.
4. Working in batches, grill them until tender.
5. Combine the 2 tablespoons of oil, balsamic vinegar, garlic, parsley, basil, and rosemary in a bowl.
6. Season with salt and pepper.
7. Drizzle the vinaigrette over the vegetables.

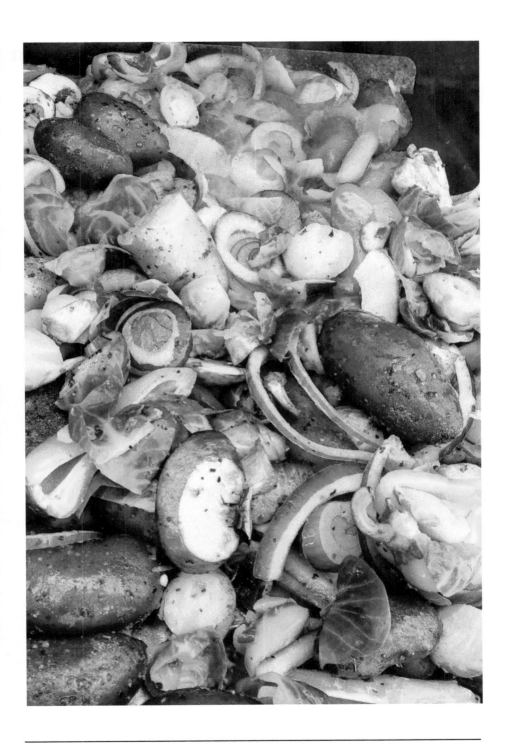

Grilled Zucchini and Red Onions in Ranch Dressing

Ingredients:

- 2 large zucchini , cut lengthwise into ½ inch slabs
- 2 large red onions, cut into ½ inch rings but don't separate into individual rings
- 2 tbsp. extra virgin olive oil
- 2 tbsp. ranch dressing mix

Directions:

1. Lightly brush each side of the vegetables with olive oil.
2. Season with the ranch dressing mix.
3. Grill over 4 minutes over medium heat or until tender.

Grilled Marinated Eggplant and Zucchini

Ingredients:

- 2 large Eggplants, cut lengthwise and cut in half
- 2 large Zucchinis, cut lengthwise and cut in half

Marinade Ingredients:

- 6 tbsp. extra virgin olive oil
- Sea salt, to taste
- 3 tbsp. distilled white vinegar
- 1 tsp. pesto sauce

Directions:

1. Marinate the vegetable with the dressing or marinade ingredients for 15 to 30 min.
2. Grill for 4 minutes over medium heat or until the vegetable becomes tender.

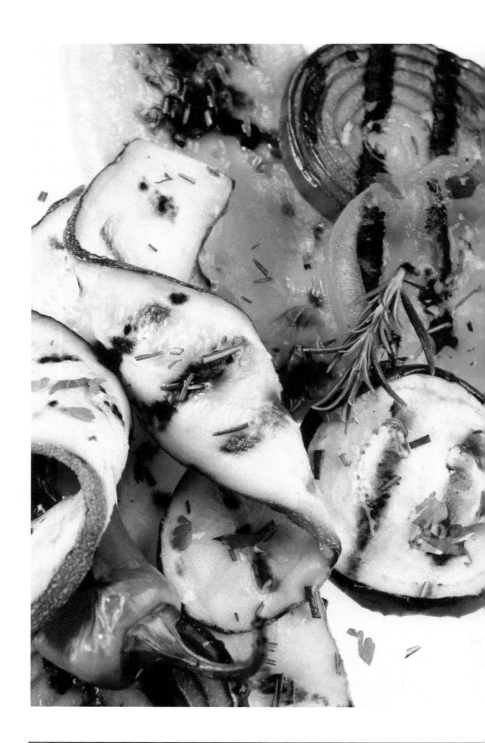

Grilled Cauliflower and Brussel Sprouts

Ingredients:

- 10 Cauliflower florets
- 10 pcs. Brussel Sprouts

Marinade Ingredients:
- 6 tbsp. extra virgin olive oil
- Sea salt, to taste
- 3 tbsp. distilled white vinegar
- 1 tsp. mayonnaise

Directions:

1. Marinate the vegetable with the dressing or marinade ingredients for 15 to 30 min.
2. Grill for 4 minutes over medium heat or until the vegetable becomes tender.

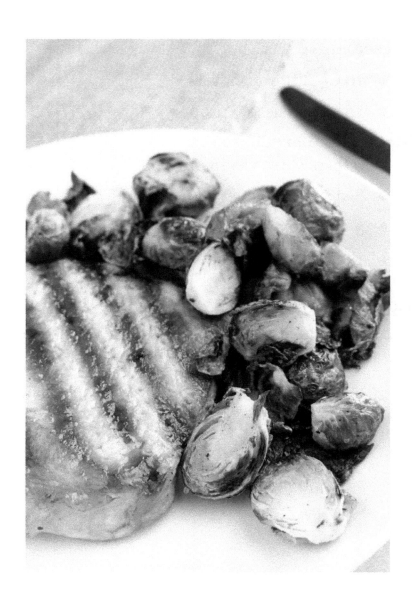

Grilled Eggplant, Zucchini and Corn

Ingredients:
- 2 large Eggplants, cut lengthwise and cut in half
- 2 large Zucchinis, cut lengthwise and cut in half
- 2 Corns, cut lengthwise

Marinade Ingredients:
- 6 tbsp. extra virgin olive oil
- Sea salt, to taste
- 3 tbsp. distilled white vinegar
- 1 tsp. mayonnaise

Directions:
1. Marinate the vegetable with the dressing or marinade ingredients for 15 to 30 min.
2. Grill for 4 minutes over medium heat or until the vegetable becomes tender.

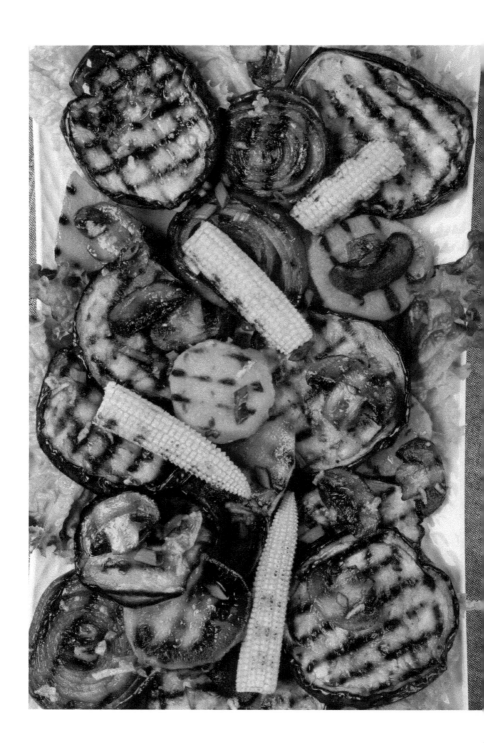

Grilled Portobello and Eggplant

Ingredients:
- 3 pcs. Portobello, rinsed and drained
- 2 pcs. Eggplant, cut lengthwise and cut in half
- 2 pcs. Zucchini, cut lengthwise and cut in half
- 6 pcs. Asparagus

Marinade Ingredients:
- 6 tbsp. extra virgin olive oil
- Sea salt, to taste
- 3 tbsp. distilled white vinegar
- 1 tsp. English mustard

Directions:
1. Marinate the vegetable with the dressing or marinade ingredients for 15 to 30 min.
2. Grill for 4 minutes over medium heat or until the vegetable becomes tender.

Grilled Japanese Eggplant and Shiitake Mushroom

Ingredients:
- Corns, cut lengthwise
- 2 pcs. Japanese Eggplant, cut lengthwise and cut in half
- 3 Shiitake Mushrooms, rinsed and drained
- Dressing Ingredients: .
- 6 tbsp. olive oil
- Sea salt, to taste
- 3 tbsp. white wine vinegar
- 1 tsp. Egg-free mayonnaise

Directions:
1. Marinate the vegetable with the dressing or marinade ingredients for 15 to 30 min.
2. Grill for 4 minutes over medium heat or until the vegetable becomes tender.

Grilled Cauliflower and Brussel Sprouts

Ingredients:
- 10 Cauliflower florets
- 10 pcs. Brussel Sprouts
- **Dressing Ingredients:**
- 6 tbsp. sesame oil
- 3 tbsp. distilled white vinegar
- 1 tsp. soy sauce
- 1 tsp. HoiSin Sauce

Directions:
1. Marinate the vegetable with the dressing or marinade ingredients for 15 to 30 min.
2. Grill for 4 minutes over medium heat or until the vegetable becomes tender.

Broccoli Florets Marinade

Ingredients:

- 6 tbsp. extra virgin olive oil

- Sea salt, to taste

- 3 tbsp. distilled white vinegar

- 1 tsp. mayonnaise

Directions:

1. Marinate the vegetable with the dressing or marinade ingredients for 15 to 30 min.

2. Grill for 4 minutes over medium heat or until the vegetable becomes tender.

Grilled Portobello Asparagus and Pineapple

Ingredients:
- 3 pcs. Portobello, rinsed and drained
- 2 pcs. Eggplant, cut lengthwise and cut in half
- 2 pcs. Zucchini, cut lengthwise and cut in half
- 6 pcs. Asparagus
- 1 medium Pineapple, cut into 1/2 inch slices
- 10 Green Beans

Dressing Ingredients:
- 6 tbsp. extra virgin olive oil
- Sea salt, to taste
- 3 tbsp. apple cider vinegar
- 1 tbsp. honey
- 1 tsp. mayonnaise

Directions:
1. Marinate the vegetable with the dressing or marinade ingredients for 15 to 30 min.
2. Grill for 4 minutes over medium heat or until the vegetable becomes tender.

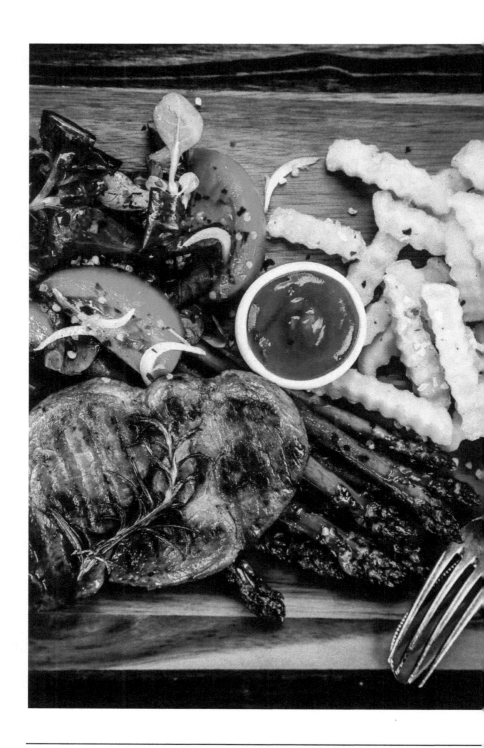

Brussel Sprouts and Endives

Ingredients:
- 10 Cauliflower florets
- 10 pcs. Brussel Sprouts
- 1 bunch of endives

Dressing Ingredients:
- 6 tbsp. olive oil
- Sea salt, to taste
- 3 tbsp. white wine vinegar
- 1 tsp. Egg-free mayonnaise

Directions:
1. Marinate the vegetable with the dressing or marinade ingredients for 15 to 30 min.
2. Grill for 4 minutes over medium heat or until the vegetable becomes tender.

Grilled Green Bean and Microgreens in Balsamic Vinaigrette

Ingredients:

- 1 bunch of microgreens
- 10 Green Beans

Dressing Ingredients:

- 6 tbsp. extra virgin olive oil
- Sea salt, to taste
- 3 tbsp. Balsamic vinegar
- 1 tsp. mustard

Directions:

1. Marinate the vegetable with the dressing or marinade ingredients for 15 to 30 min.
2. Grill for 4 minutes over medium heat or until the vegetable becomes tender.

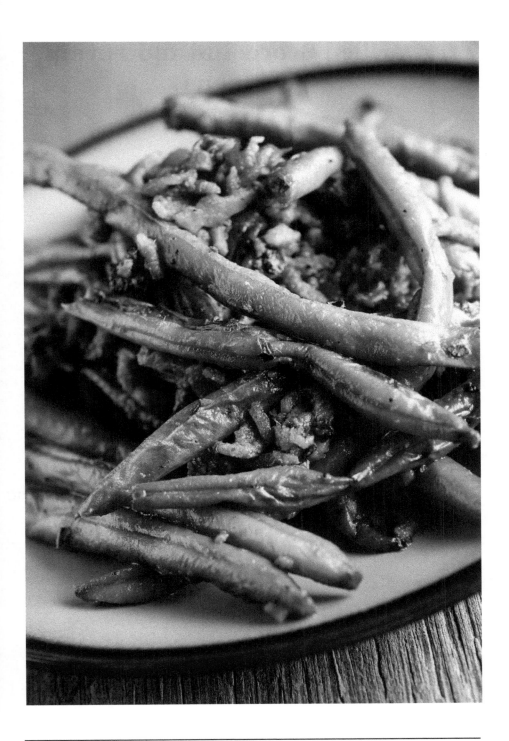

Grilled Broccolini and Turnip Greens

Ingredients:
- 1 bunch of turnip greens
- 8 Broccolini Florets

Dressing Ingredients:
- 6 tbsp. sesame oil
- Sea salt, to taste
- 3 tbsp. distilled white vinegar
- 1 tsp. Egg-free mayonnaise

Directions:
1. Marinate the vegetable with the dressing or marinade ingredients for 15 to 30 min.
2. Grill for 4 minutes over medium heat or until the vegetable becomes tender.

Grilled Green Cabbage in Apple Cider Vinaigrette

Ingredients:
- 1 large parsnip, peeled and cut lengthwise
- 5 pcs. Portobello mushrooms, rinsed and drained
- 1 Green cabbage, cut in half

Dressing Ingredients:
- 6 tbsp. extra virgin olive oil
- Sea salt, to taste
- 3 tbsp. apple cider vinegar
- 1 tbsp. honey
- 1 tsp. Egg-free mayonnaise

Directions:
1. Marinate the vegetable with the dressing or marinade ingredients for 15 to 30 min.
2. Grill for 4 minutes over medium heat or until the vegetable becomes tender.

Grilled Parsnip and Rutabaga

Ingredients:
- 1 large parsnip, peeled and cut lengthwise
- 1 medium Rutabaga, peeled and cut in half lengthwise
- 2 large red onions, cut into ½ inch rings but don't separate into individual rings

Marinade Ingredients:
- 6 tbsp. extra virgin olive oil
- Sea salt, to taste
- 3 tbsp. distilled white vinegar
- 1 tsp. Dijon mustard

Directions:
1. Marinate the vegetable with the dressing or marinade ingredients for 15 to 30 min.
2. Grill for 4 minutes over medium heat or until the vegetable becomes tender.

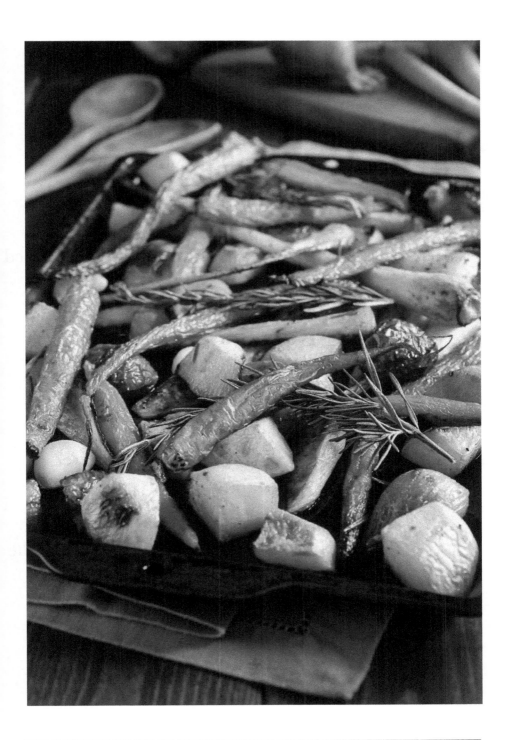

Grilled Carrot, Turnip and Water Chestnuts with Balsamic Glaze

Ingredients:
- 1 large carrots, peeled and cut lengthwise
- 1 large turnip, peeled and cut lengthwise
- 1/2 cup canned water chestnuts
- 2 pcs. Portobello mushrooms, rinsed and drained

Dressing Ingredients:
- 6 tbsp. extra virgin olive oil
- Sea salt, to taste
- 3 tbsp. Balsamic vinegar
- 1 tsp. Dijon mustard

Directions:
1. Marinate the vegetable with the dressing or marinade ingredients for 15 to 30 min.
2. Grill for 4 minutes over medium heat or until the vegetable becomes tender

Grilled beetroots and Green Beans

Ingredients:

- 2 beetroots, peeled and sliced lengthwise
- 1 medium Pineapple, cut into 1/2 inch slices
- 10 Green Beans
- 2 large red onions, cut into ½ inch rings but don't separate into individual rings

Dressing Ingredients:

- 6 tbsp. olive oil
- Sea salt, to taste
- 3 tbsp. white wine vinegar
- 1 tsp. English mustard

Directions:

1. Marinate the vegetable with the dressing or marinade ingredients for 15 to 30 min.
2. Grill for 4 minutes over medium heat or until the vegetable becomes tender.

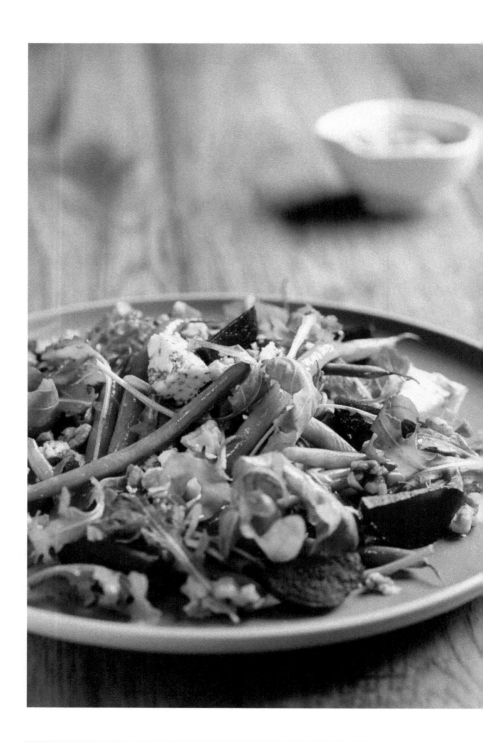

Grilles Turnips Broccolini and Water Chestnuts with Honey Apple Cider Glaze

Ingredients:
- 10 Broccolini Florets
- 1/2 cup water chestnuts
- 1 large turnip, peeled and cut lengthwise

Dressing Ingredients:
- 6 tbsp. extra virgin olive oil
- Sea salt, to taste
- 3 tbsp. apple cider vinegar
- 1 tbsp. honey
- 1 tsp. Egg-free mayonnaise

Directions:
1. Marinate the vegetable with the dressing or marinade ingredients for 15 to 30 min.
2. Grill for 4 minutes over medium heat or until the vegetable becomes tender.

Grilled Eggplant & Beetroot with Assorted Bell Peppers

Ingredients:

- 1 small Eggplant, cut lengthwise and cut in half
- 2 beetroots, peeled and sliced lengthwise
- 1 large turnip, peeled and cut lengthwise
- 1 Yellow Bell Pepper, cut in half
- 1 Red Bell Pepper, cut in half

Dressing Ingredients:

- 6 tbsp. sesame oil
- Sea salt, to taste
- 3 tbsp. distilled white vinegar
- 1 tsp. Egg-free mayonnaise

Directions:

1. Marinate the vegetable with the dressing or marinade ingredients for 15 to 30 min.
2. Grill for 4 minutes over medium heat or until the vegetable becomes tender.

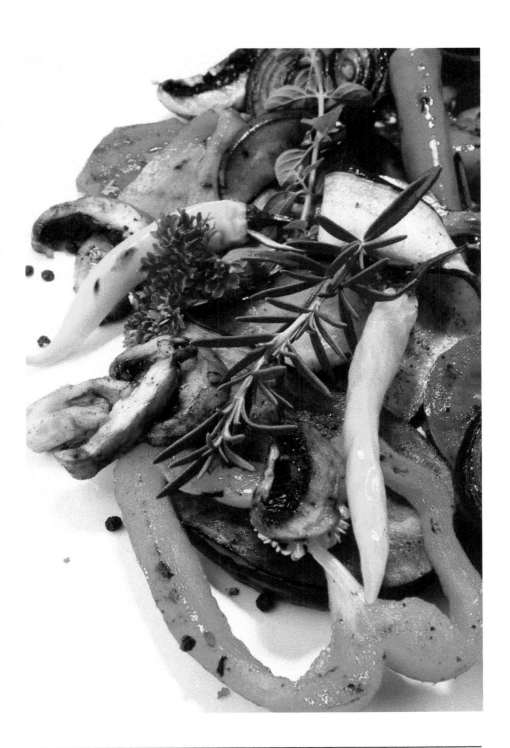

Grilled Water Chestnuts Zucchini and Endives

Ingredients:
- 2 large zucchini , cut lengthwise into ½ inch slabs
- 1/2 cup water chestnuts
- 1 bunch of endives

Dressing Ingredients:
- 6 tbsp. sesame oil
- Sea salt, to taste
- 3 tbsp. distilled white vinegar
- 1 tsp. Egg-free mayonnaise

Directions:
1. Marinate the vegetable with the dressing or marinade ingredients for 15 to 30 min.
2. Grill for 4 minutes over medium heat or until the vegetable becomes tender.

Grilled Collard Greens Portobello and Asparagus

Ingredients:
- 3 pcs. Portobello, rinsed and drained
- 1 medium Rutabaga, peeled and cut in half lengthwise
- 1 bunch of collard greens
- 6 pcs. Asparagus

Dressing Ingredients:
- 6 tbsp. sesame oil
- Sea salt, to taste
- 3 tbsp. distilled white vinegar
- 1 tsp. Egg-free mayonnaise

Directions:
1. Marinate the vegetable with the dressing or marinade ingredients for 15 to 30 min.
2. Grill for 4 minutes over medium heat or until the vegetable becomes tender.

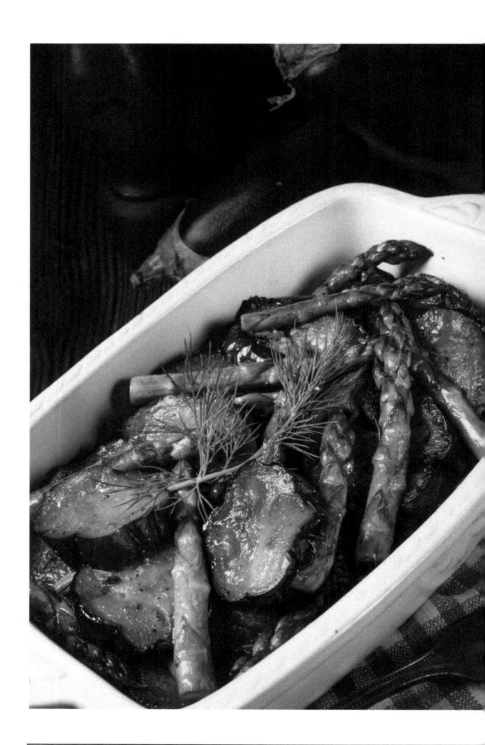

Grilled Rutabaga and Swiss Chard

Ingredients:

- medium Rutabaga, peeled and cut in half lengthwise
- 2 large red onions, cut into ½ inch rings but don't separate into individual rings
- 1 bunch of swiss chard

Marinade Ingredients:

- 6 tbsp. extra virgin olive oil
- Sea salt, to taste
- 3 tbsp. distilled white vinegar
- 1 tsp. Dijon mustard

Directions:

1. Marinate the vegetable with the dressing or marinade ingredients for 15 to 30 min.
2. Grill for 4 minutes over medium heat or until the vegetable becomes tender.

Grilled Green Beans and Eggplants

Ingredients:
- 2 beetroots, peeled and sliced lengthwise
- 2 large Zucchinis, cut lengthwise and cut in half
- 10 Green Beans

Dressing Ingredients:
- 6 tbsp. extra virgin olive oil
- Sea salt, to taste
- 3 tbsp. Balsamic vinegar
- 1 tsp. Dijon mustard

Directions:
1. Marinate the vegetable with the dressing or marinade ingredients for 15 to 30 min.
2. Grill for 4 minutes over medium heat or until the vegetable becomes tender.

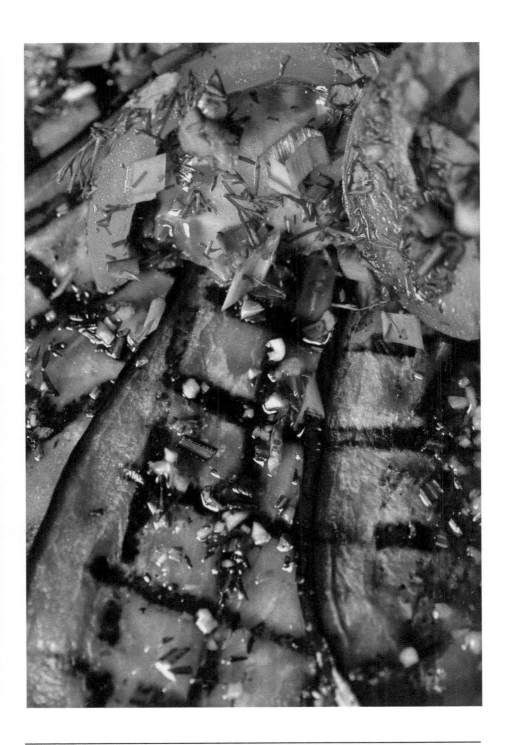

Grilled Collard Greens and Brussel Sprouts

Ingredients:
- 1 bunch of collard greens
- 10 pcs. Brussel Sprouts
- 10 Broccolini Florets
- 1 bunch of swiss chard

Dressing Ingredients:
- 6 tbsp. olive oil
- Sea salt, to taste
- 3 tbsp. white wine vinegar
- 1 tsp. English mustard

Directions:
1. Marinate the vegetable with the dressing or marinade ingredients for 15 to 30 min.
2. Grill for 4 minutes over medium heat or until the vegetable becomes tender.

Grilled Swiss Chard and Asparagus

Ingredients:

- 1 medium Rutabaga, peeled and cut in half lengthwise
- 2 large red onions, cut into ½ inch rings but don't separate into individual rings
- 1 bunch of swiss chard
- 10 pcs. Asparagus

Dressing Ingredients:

- 6 tbsp. extra virgin olive oil
- Sea salt, to taste
- 3 tbsp. apple cider vinegar
- 1 tbsp. honey
- 1 tsp. Egg-free mayonnaise

Directions:

1. Marinate the vegetable with the dressing or marinade ingredients for 15 to 30 min.
2. Grill for 4 minutes over medium heat or until the vegetable becomes tender.

Grilled Endives and Edamame Beans

Ingredients:

- 10 Edamame Beans

- 2 beetroots, peeled and sliced lengthwise

- 1 bunch of endives

Dressing Ingredients:

- 6 tbsp. olive oil

- Sea salt, to taste

- 3 tbsp. white wine vinegar

- 1 tsp. Egg-free mayonnaise

Directions:

1. Marinate the vegetable with the dressing or marinade ingredients for 15 to 30 min.

2. Grill for 4 minutes over medium heat or until the vegetable becomes tender.

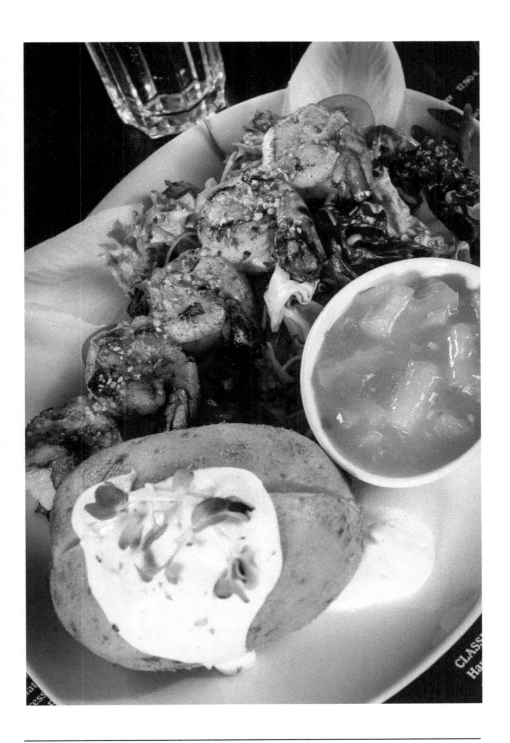

Grilled Water Chestnuts and Cabbage

Ingredients:
- 1 Green cabbage
- 1/2 cup water chestnuts
- 2 large red onions, cut into ½ inch rings but don't separate into individual rings
- 2 tbsp. extra virgin olive oil
- 2 tbsp. ranch dressing mix

Directions:
1. Marinate the vegetable with the dressing or marinade ingredients for 15 to 30 min.
2. Grill for 4 minutes over medium heat or until the vegetable becomes tender.

Grilled Okra and Water Chestnuts

Ingredients:
- 1 Red cabbage
- 1/2 cup water chestnuts
- 5 pcs. Okra
- 3 pcs. Asparagus Corns, cut lengthwise
- 2 pcs. Portobello mushrooms, rinsed and drained

Marinade Ingredients:
- 6 tbsp. extra virgin olive oil
- Sea salt, to taste
- 3 tbsp. distilled white vinegar
- 1 tsp. Dijon mustard

Directions:
1. Marinate the vegetable with the dressing or marinade ingredients for 15 to 30 min.
2. Grill for 4 minutes over medium heat or until the vegetable becomes tender.

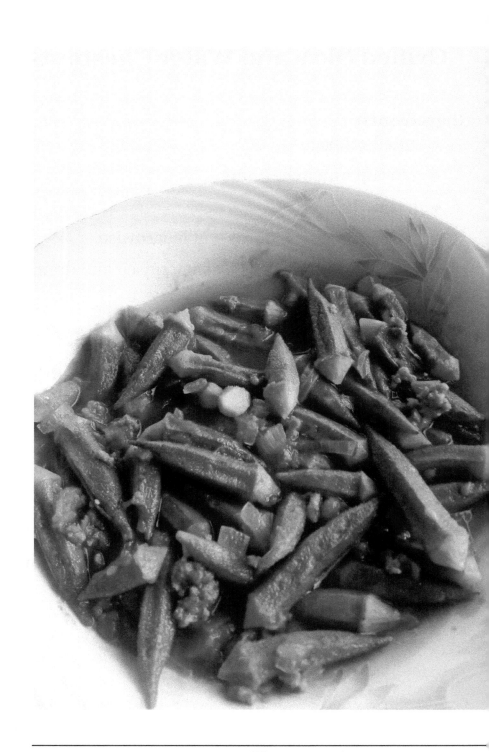

Grilled Turnip Greens and Broccolini

Ingredients:
- 1 bunch of turnip greens
- 10 pcs. Brussel Sprouts
- 10 Broccolini Florets
- 10 pcs. Asparagus

Dressing Ingredients:
- 6 tbsp. sesame oil
- Sea salt, to taste
- 3 tbsp. distilled white vinegar
- 1 tsp. Egg-free mayonnaise

Directions:
1. Marinate the vegetable with the dressing or marinade ingredients for 15 to 30 min.
2. Grill for 4 minutes over medium heat or until the vegetable becomes tender.

Grilled Parsnip and Microgreens

Ingredients:
- 1 large Parsnip, cut lengthwise
- 1 bunch of microgreens
- 2 large red onions, cut into ½ inch rings but don't separate into individual rings

Dressing Ingredients:
- 6 tbsp. olive oil
- Sea salt, to taste
- 3 tbsp. white wine vinegar
- 1 tsp. Egg-free mayonnaise

Directions:
1. Marinate the vegetable with the dressing or marinade ingredients for 15 to 30 min.
2. Grill for 4 minutes over medium heat or until the vegetable becomes tender.

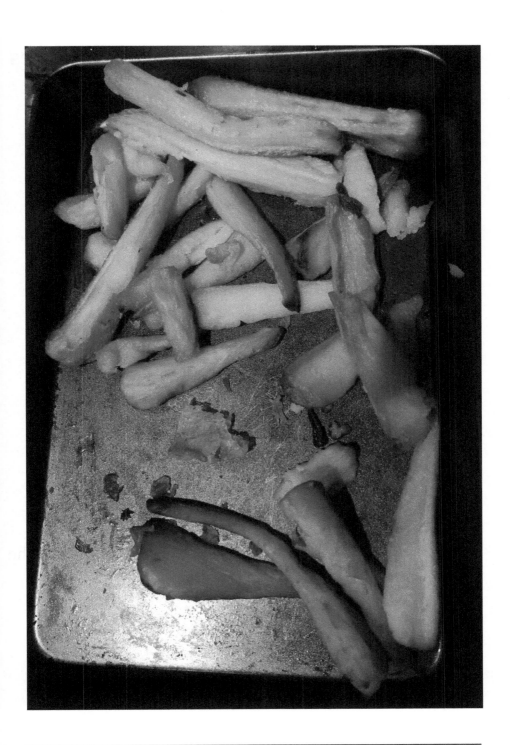

Grilled Carrot, Parsnip and Endives

Ingredients:
- 1 large Carrot, cut lengthwise
- 1 large Parsnip, cut lengthwise
- 1 bunch of endives
- 10 pcs. Asparagus
- 10 Green Beans

Dressing Ingredients:
- 6 tbsp. olive oil
- Sea salt, to taste
- 3 tbsp. white wine vinegar
- 1 tsp.English mustard

Directions:
1. Marinate the vegetable with the dressing or marinade ingredients for 15 to 30 min.
2. Grill for 4 minutes over medium heat or until the vegetable becomes tender.

Grilled Cauliflower and Baby Corn

Ingredients:
- 10 Cauliflower florets ½ cup canned baby corn
- 10 pcs. Brussel Sprouts

Dressing Ingredients:
- 6 tbsp. extra virgin olive oil
- Sea salt, to taste
- 3 tbsp. apple cider vinegar
- 1 tbsp. honey
- 1 tsp. Egg-free mayonnaise

Directions:
1. Marinate the vegetable with the dressing or marinade ingredients for 15 to 30 min.
2. Grill for 4 minutes over medium heat or until the vegetable becomes tender.

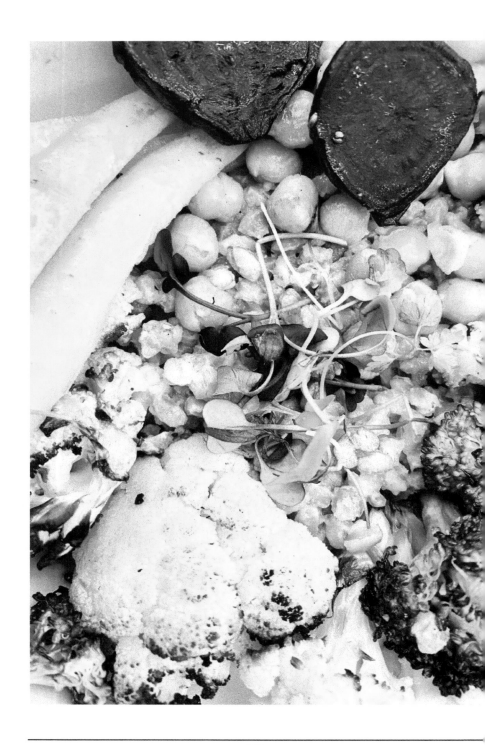

Grilled Baby Carrots and Beetroots

Ingredients:
- 5 pcs. baby carrots
- 2 large Eggplants, cut lengthwise and cut in half
- 2 beetroots, peeled and sliced lengthwise

Dressing Ingredients:
- 6 tbsp. sesame oil
- Sea salt, to taste
- 3 tbsp. distilled white vinegar
- 1 tsp. Egg-free mayonnaise

Directions:
1. Marinate the vegetable with the dressing or marinade ingredients for 15 to 30 min.
2. Grill for 4 minutes over medium heat or until the vegetable becomes tender.

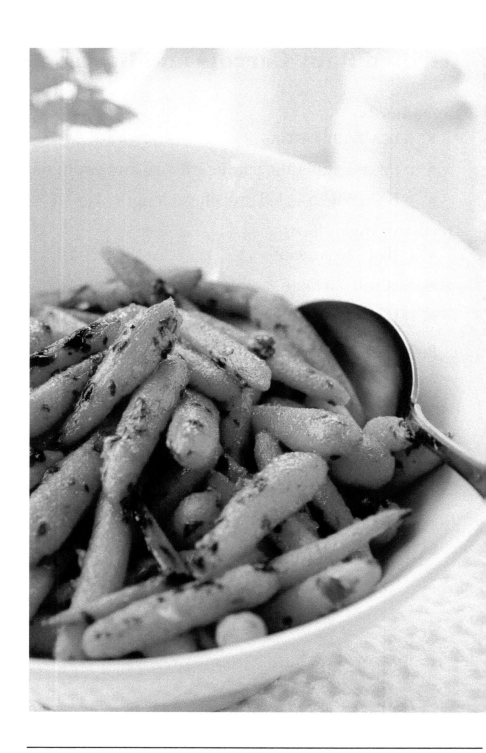

Grilled Microgreens and Beetroots

Ingredients:
- 1 bunch of microgreens
- 2 beetroots, peeled and sliced lengthwise
- Corns, cut lengthwise

Dressing Ingredients:
- 6 tbsp. extra virgin olive oil
- Sea salt, to taste
- 3 tbsp. Balsamic vinegar
- 1 tsp. Dijon mustard

Directions:
1. Marinate the vegetable with the dressing or marinade ingredients for 15 to 30 min.
2. Grill for 4 minutes over medium heat or until the vegetable becomes tender.

Grilled Rutabaga Pineapple and Artichoke Hearts

Ingredients:
- 1 medium Pineapple, cut into 1/2 inch slices
- 1 medium Rutabaga, peeled and cut in half lengthwise
- 1 cup canned artichoke hearts

Marinade Ingredients:
- 6 tbsp. extra virgin olive oil
- Sea salt, to taste
- 3 tbsp. distilled white vinegar
- 1 tsp. Dijon mustard

Directions:
1. Marinate the vegetable with the dressing or marinade ingredients for 15 to 30 min.
2. Grill for 4 minutes over medium heat or until the vegetable becomes tender.

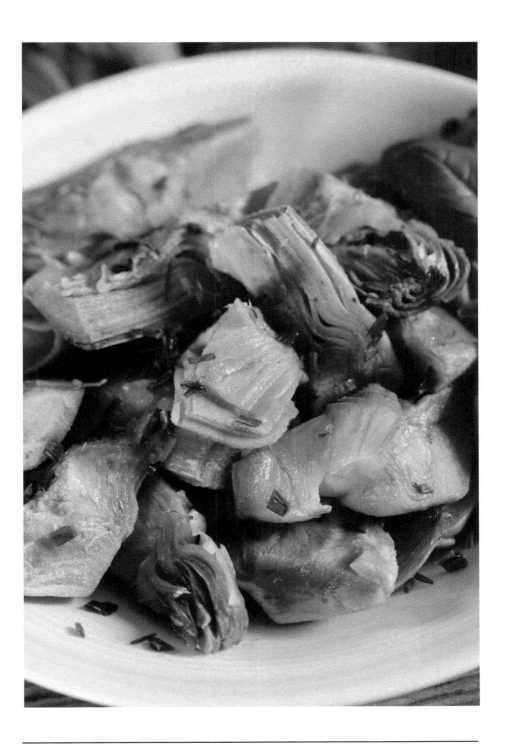

Simple Grilled Water Chestnuts and Cauliflower Florets

Ingredients:
- 1/2 cup canned water chestnuts
- 10 Cauliflower florets
- 10 pcs. Brussel Sprouts

Dressing Ingredients:
- 6 tbsp. extra virgin olive oil
- Sea salt, to taste
- 3 tbsp. apple cider vinegar
- 1 tbsp. honey
- 1 tsp. Egg-free mayonnaise

Directions:
1. Marinate the vegetable with the dressing or marinade ingredients for 15 to 30 min.
2. Grill for 4 minutes over medium heat or until the vegetable becomes tender.

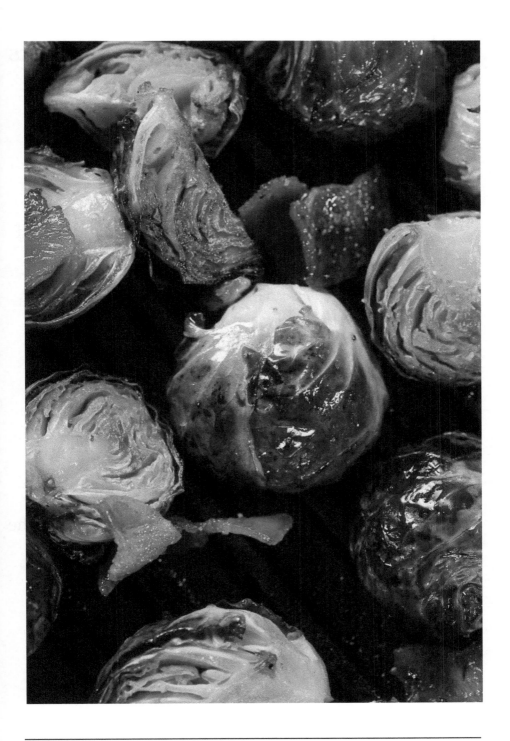

Grilled Baby Corn, Water Chestnuts and Eggplant

Ingredients:
- 1/2 cup canned baby corn
- 1/2 cup canned water chestnuts
- 2 large Eggplants, cut lengthwise and cut in half

Dressing Ingredients:
- 6 tbsp. olive oil
- Sea salt, to taste
- 3 tbsp. white wine vinegar
- 1 tsp. Egg-free mayonnaise

Directions:
1. Marinate the vegetable with the dressing or marinade ingredients for 15 to 30 min.
2. Grill for 4 minutes over medium heat or until the vegetable becomes tender.

Grilled Broccolini Beetroots and Portobello Mushroom

Ingredients:
- 10 Broccolini Florets
- 2 beetroots, peeled and sliced lengthwise
- Corns, cut lengthwise
- 5 pcs. Portobello mushrooms, rinsed and drained

Dressing Ingredients:
- 6 tbsp. sesame oil
- Sea salt, to taste
- 3 tbsp. distilled white vinegar
- 1 tsp. Egg-free mayonnaise

Directions:
1. Marinate the vegetable with the dressing or marinade ingredients for 15 to 30 min.
2. Grill for 4 minutes over medium heat or until the vegetable becomes tender.

Grilled Baby Carrots and Baby Carrots

Ingredients:
- 10 pcs. Baby Carrots
- 2 beetroots, peeled and sliced lengthwise

Dressing Ingredients:
- 6 tbsp. olive oil
- Sea salt, to taste
- 3 tbsp. white wine vinegar
- 1 tsp. Egg-free mayonnaise

Directions:
1. Marinate the vegetable with the dressing or marinade ingredients for 15 to 30 min.
2. Grill for 4 minutes over medium heat or until the vegetable becomes tender.

Grilled Turnip Greens

Ingredients:

- 1 bunch of turnip greens

Dressing Ingredients:

- 6 tbsp. olive oil

- Sea salt, to taste

- 3 tbsp. white wine vinegar

- 1 tsp. Egg-free mayonnaise

Directions:

1. Marinate the vegetable with the dressing or marinade ingredients for 15 to 30 min.

2. Grill for 4 minutes over medium heat or until the vegetable becomes tender.

Grilled Broccolini Florets and Summer Squash

Ingredients:
- 10 Broccolini Florets
- 10 pcs. Brussel Sprouts
- 10 pcs. Asparagus
- 1 summer squash, peeled and sliced lengthwise
- 4 large Tomatoes, sliced thick

Dressing Ingredients:
- 6 tbsp. extra virgin olive oil
- 1 tsp. onion powder
- Sea salt, to taste
- 3 tbsp. distilled white vinegar
- 1 tsp. Dijon mustard

Directions:
1. Combine all of the dressing ingredients thoroughly.
2. Preheat your grill to low heat and grease the grates.

3. Layer the vegetables grill for 12 minutes per side, until tender flipping once.
4. Brush with the marinade/ dressing ingredients

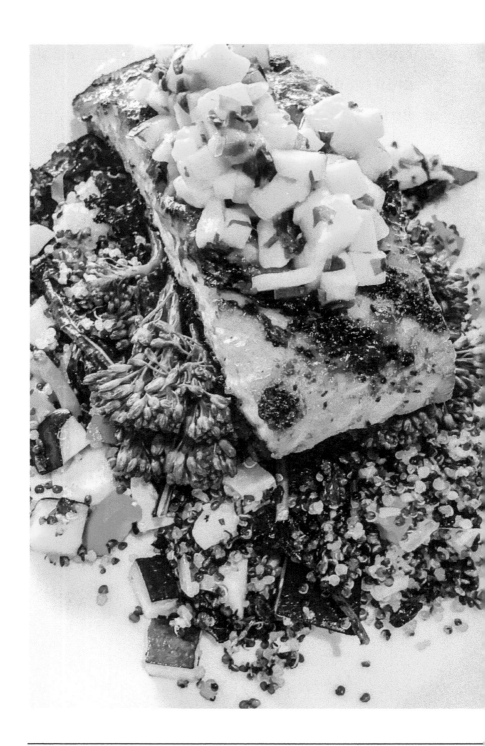

Grilled Winter Squash and Eggplant

Ingredients:
- 1 lb eggplant, sliced lengthwise into shorter sticks
- 1 winter squash, peeled and sliced lengthwise
- 1 large red onion, cut into 1/2 inch thick rounds
- 1/3 cup Italian parsley or basil, finely chopped

Dressing Ingredients:
- 6 tbsp. extra virgin olive oil
- 1 tsp. onion powder
- Sea salt, to taste
- 3 tbsp. distilled white vinegar
- 1 tsp. Dijon mustard

Directions:
1. Combine all of the dressing ingredients thoroughly.
2. Preheat your grill to low heat and grease the grates.
3. Layer the vegetables grill for 12 minutes per side, until tender flipping once.
4. Brush with the marinade/ dressing ingredients

Grilled Zucchini and Green Bell Peppers

Ingredients:
- 1 lb zucchini, sliced lengthwise into shorter sticks
- 1 lb green bell peppers, sliced into wide strips
- 1 large red onion, cut into 1/2 inch thick rounds
- 1/3 cup Italian parsley or basil, finely chopped

Dressing Ingredients:
- 6 tbsp. extra virgin olive oil
- Sea salt, to taste
- 3 tbsp. apple cider vinegar
- 1 tbsp. honey
- 1 tsp. Egg-free mayonnaise

Directions:
1. Combine all of the dressing ingredients thoroughly.
2. Preheat your grill to low heat and grease the grates.
3. Layer the vegetables grill for 12 minutes per side, until tender flipping once.
4. Brush with the marinade/ dressing ingredients

Grilled Zucchini & Butternut Squash

Ingredients:
- 1 lb zucchini, sliced lengthwise into shorter sticks
- 1 butternut squash, peeled and sliced len
- 1 large red onion, cut into 1/2 inch thick rounds
- 1/3 cup Italian parsley or basil, finely chopped

Dressing Ingredients:
- 6 tbsp. olive oil
- 1 tsp. garlic powder
- 1 tsp. onion powder
- Sea salt, to taste
- 3 tbsp. white wine vinegar
- 1 tsp. English mustard

Directions:
1. Combine all of the dressing ingredients thoroughly.
2. Preheat your grill to low heat and grease the grates.
3. Layer the vegetables grill for 12 minutes per side, until tender flipping once.
4. Brush with the marinade/ dressing ingredients

Grilled Baby Corn Zucchini and Beetroots

Ingredients:
- 1/2 cup baby corn
- 1 lb zucchini, sliced lengthwise into shorter sticks
- 2 beetroots, peeled and sliced lengthwise
- 1 large red onion, cut into 1/2 inch thick rounds
- 1/3 cup Italian parsley or basil, finely chopped

Dressing Ingredients:
- 6 tbsp. olive oil
- 3 dashes of Tabasco hot sauce
- Sea salt, to taste
- 3 tbsp. white wine vinegar
- 1 tsp. Egg-free mayonnaise

Directions:
1. Combine all of the dressing ingredients thoroughly.
2. Preheat your grill to low heat and grease the grates.

3. Layer the vegetables grill for 12 minutes per side, until tender flipping once.
4. Brush with the marinade/ dressing ingredients

Grilled Summer Squash and Carrots

Ingredients:
- 1 summer squash, peeled and sliced lengthwise
- 1 baby carrots, rinsed
- 1 large red onion, cut into 1/2 inch thick rounds
- 1/3 cup Italian parsley or basil, finely chopped

Dressing Ingredients:
- 6 tbsp. extra virgin olive oil
- Sea salt, to taste
- 3 tbsp. Balsamic vinegar
- 1 tsp. Dijon mustard

Directions:
1. Combine all of the dressing ingredients thoroughly.
2. Preheat your grill to low heat and grease the grates.
3. Layer the vegetables grill for 12 minutes per side, until tender flipping once.
4. Brush with the marinade/ dressing ingredients.

Grilled Edamame Beans and Zucchini

Ingredients:
- 20 pcs. Edamame Beans
- 1 lb zucchini, sliced lengthwise into shorter sticks
- 1 lb green bell peppers, sliced into wide strips
- 1 large red onion, cut into 1/2 inch thick rounds
- 1/3 cup Italian parsley or basil, finely chopped

Dressing Ingredients:
- 6 tbsp. extra virgin olive oil
- 1 tsp. onion powder
- Sea salt, to taste
- 3 tbsp. distilled white vinegar
- 1 tsp. Dijon mustard

Directions:
1. Combine all of the dressing ingredients thoroughly.
2. Preheat your grill to low heat and grease the grates.

3. Layer the vegetables grill for 12 minutes per side, until tender flipping once.
4. Brush with the marinade/ dressing ingredients

Grilled Okra and Mustard Greens

Ingredients:
- 10 pcs. Okra
- 1 bunch of mustard greens
- 10 pcs. Brussel Sprouts
- 1 large red onion, cut into 1/2 inch thick rounds
- 1/3 cup Italian parsley or basil, finely chopped

Dressing Ingredients:
- 6 tbsp. olive oil
- 3 dashes of Tabasco hot sauce
- Sea salt, to taste
- 3 tbsp. white wine vinegar
- 1 tsp. Egg-free mayonnaise

Directions:
1. Combine all of the dressing ingredients thoroughly.
2. Preheat your grill to low heat and grease the grates.
3. Layer the vegetables grill for 12 minutes per side, until tender flipping once.
4. Brush with the marinade/ dressing ingredients

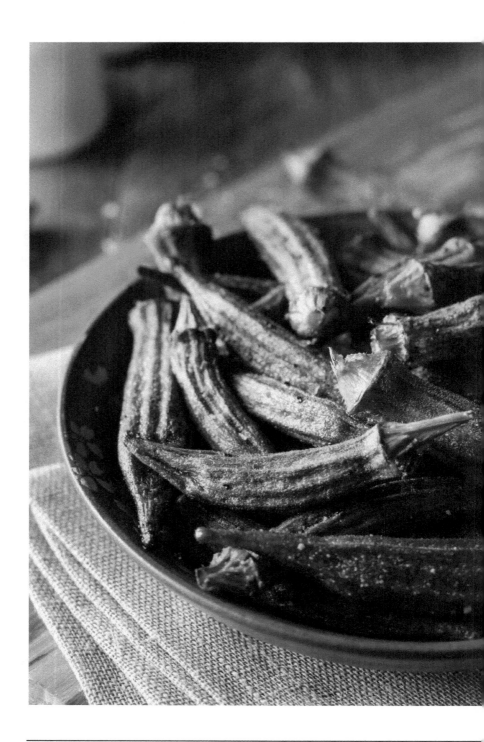

Grilled Beetroots & Kale

Ingredients:
- 1 bunch of Kale
- 2 beetroots, peeled and sliced lengthwise
- 1/3 cup Italian parsley or basil, finely chopped

Dressing Ingredients:
- 6 tbsp. extra virgin olive oil
- Sea salt, to taste
- 1 tsp. onion powder
- 1/2 tsp. Herbs de Provence
- 3 tbsp. white vinegar
- 1 tsp. Dijon mustard

Directions:
1. Combine all of the dressing ingredients thoroughly.
2. Preheat your grill to low heat and grease the grates.
3. Layer the vegetables grill for 12 minutes per side, until tender flipping once.
4. Brush with the marinade/ dressing ingredients.

Grilled Edamame Beans and Summer Squash

Ingredients:
- 20 pcs. Edamame Beans
- 1 bunch of Romaine Lettuce leaves
- 1 summer squash, peeled and sliced lengthwise
- 4 large Tomatoes, sliced thick

Dressing Ingredients:
- 6 tbsp. extra virgin olive oil
- 1 tsp. onion powder
- Sea salt, to taste
- 3 tbsp. distilled white vinegar
- 1 tsp. Dijon mustard

Directions:
1. Combine all of the dressing ingredients thoroughly.
2. Preheat your grill to low heat and grease the grates.
3. Layer the vegetables grill for 12 minutes per side, until tender flipping once.
4. Brush with the marinade/ dressing ingredients.

Grilled Beetroots and Broccolini

Ingredients:
- 2 beetroots, peeled and sliced lengthwise
- 1 large red onion, cut into 1/2 inch thick rounds
- 1/3 cup Italian parsley or basil, finely chopped
- 10 Broccolini Florets
- 10 pcs. Brussel Sprouts

Dressing Ingredients:
- 6 tbsp. olive oil
- 3 dashes of Tabasco hot sauce
- Sea salt, to taste
- 3 tbsp. white wine vinegar
- 1 tsp. Egg-free mayonnaise

Directions:
1. Combine all of the dressing ingredients thoroughly.
2. Preheat your grill to low heat and grease the grates.
3. Layer the vegetables grill for 12 minutes per side, until tender flipping once.
4. Brush with the marinade/ dressing ingredients.

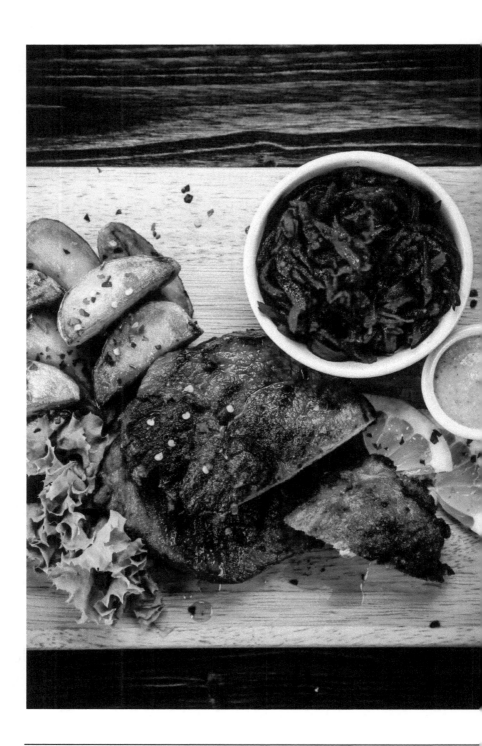

Grilled Artichokes and Mustard Greens

Ingredients:
- 1 pc. Artichoke
- 1 bunch of mustard greens
- 1/3 cup Italian parsley or basil, finely chopped

Dressing Ingredients:
- 6 tbsp. extra virgin olive oil
- Sea salt, to taste
- 3 tbsp. apple cider vinegar
- 1 tbsp. honey
- 1 tsp. Egg-free mayonnaise

Directions:
1. Combine all of the dressing ingredients thoroughly.
2. Preheat your grill to low heat and grease the grates.
3. Layer the vegetables grill for 12 minutes per side, until tender flipping once.
4. Brush with the marinade/ dressing ingredients.

Grilled Beets and Swiss Chard

Ingredients:

- 5 pcs. Beets
- 1 bunch of swiss chard
- 4 large Tomatoes, sliced thick
- 1/3 cup Italian parsley or basil, finely chopped

Dressing Ingredients:

- 6 tbsp. extra virgin olive oil
- 1 tsp. onion powder
- Sea salt, to taste
- 3 tbsp. distilled white vinegar
- 1 tsp. Dijon mustard

Directions:

1. Combine all of the dressing ingredients thoroughly.
2. Preheat your grill to low heat and grease the grates.
3. Layer the vegetables grill for 12 minutes per side, until tender flipping once.
4. Brush with the marinade/ dressing ingredients.

Grilled Baby Corn and Winter Squash

Ingredients:

- 10 pcs. baby corn
- 1 winter squash, peeled and sliced lengthwise
- 1 large red onion, cut into 1/2 inch thick rounds
- 1/3 cup Italian parsley or basil, finely chopped

Dressing Ingredients:

- 6 tbsp. olive oil
- 3 dashes of Tabasco hot sauce
- Sea salt, to taste
- 3 tbsp. white wine vinegar
- 1 tsp. Egg-free mayonnaise

Directions:

1. Combine all of the dressing ingredients thoroughly.
2. Preheat your grill to low heat and grease the grates.

3. Layer the vegetables grill for 12 minutes per side, until tender flipping once.
4. Brush with the marinade/ dressing ingredients.

Grilled Beets and Asparagus

Ingredients:

- 5 pcs. Beets
- 10 pcs. Asparagus
- 1 winter squash, peeled and sliced lengthwise
- 4 large Tomatoes, sliced thick
- 1 lb green bell peppers, sliced into wide strips
- 1 large red onion, cut into 1/2 inch thick rounds
- 1/3 cup Italian parsley or basil, finely chopped

Dressing Ingredients:

- 6 tbsp. extra virgin olive oil
- Sea salt, to taste .
- 3 tbsp. apple cider vinegar
- 1 tbsp. honey
- 1 tsp. Egg-free mayonnaise

Directions:

1. Combine all of the dressing ingredients thoroughly.
2. Preheat your grill to low heat and grease the grates.

3. Layer the vegetables grill for 12 minutes per side, until tender flipping once.
4. Brush with the marinade/ dressing ingredients

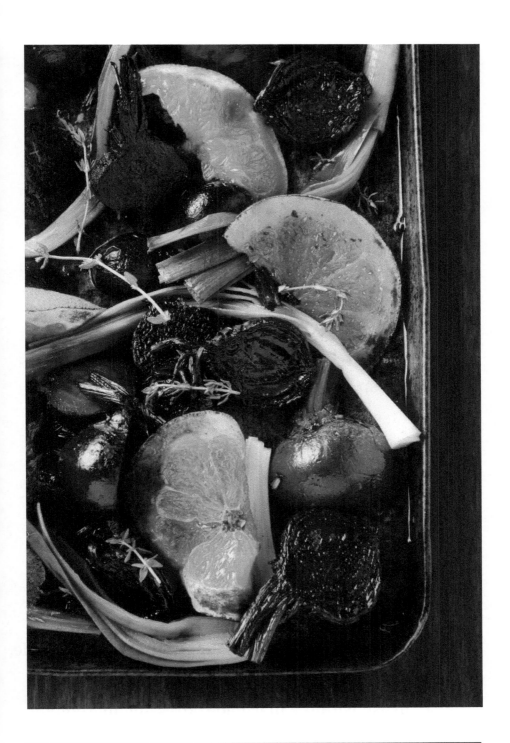

Grilled Artichoke

Ingredients:

- 1 pc. Artichoke
- 1/3 cup Italian parsley or basil, finely chopped

Dressing Ingredients:

- 6 tbsp. extra virgin olive oil
- 1 tsp. onion powder
- Sea salt, to taste
- 3 tbsp. distilled white vinegar
- 1 tsp. Dijon mustard

Directions:

1. Combine all of the dressing ingredients thoroughly.
2. Preheat your grill to low heat and grease the grates.
3. Layer the vegetables grill for 12 minutes per side, until tender flipping once.
4. Brush with the marinade/ dressing ingredients.

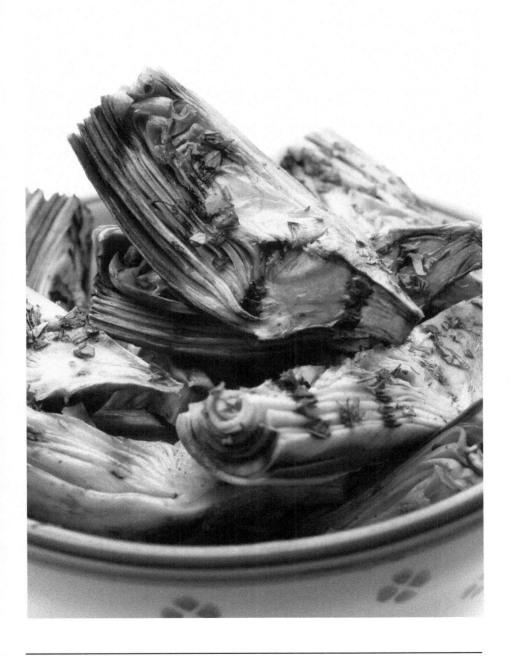

Grilled Summer Squash Cabbage and Romaine Lettuce

Ingredients:

- 1 medium Cabbage sliced
- 1 summer squash, peeled and sliced lengthwise
- 4 large Tomatoes, sliced thick
- 1 large red onion, cut into 1/2 inch thick rounds
- 1/3 cup Italian parsley or basil, finely chopped

Dressing Ingredients:

- 6 tbsp. olive oil
- 3 dashes of Tabasco hot sauce
- Sea salt, to taste
- 3 tbsp. white wine vinegar
- 1 tsp. Egg-free mayonnaise

Directions:

1. Combine all of the dressing ingredients thoroughly.

2. Preheat your grill to low heat and grease the grates.
3. Layer the vegetables grill for 12 minutes per side, until tender flipping once.
4. Brush with the marinade/ dressing ingredients.

Grilled Rutabaga Baby Carrots and Brussels Sprouts

Ingredients:

- 8 pcs. baby carrots
- 1 lb green bell peppers, sliced into wide strips
- 1 medium Rutabaga, peeled and cut in half lengthwise
- 10 pcs. Brussel Sprouts
- 1 large red onion, cut into 1/2 inch thick rounds
- 1/3 cup Italian parsley or basil, finely chopped

Dressing Ingredients:

- 6 tbsp. extra virgin olive oil
- Sea salt, to taste
- 1 tsp. onion powder
- 1/2 tsp. Herbs de Provence
- 3 tbsp. white vinegar
- 1 tsp.Dijon mustard

Directions:

1. Combine all of the dressing ingredients thoroughly.
2. Preheat your grill to low heat and grease the grates.

3. Layer the vegetables grill for 12 minutes per side, until tender flipping once.
4. Brush with the marinade/ dressing ingredients.

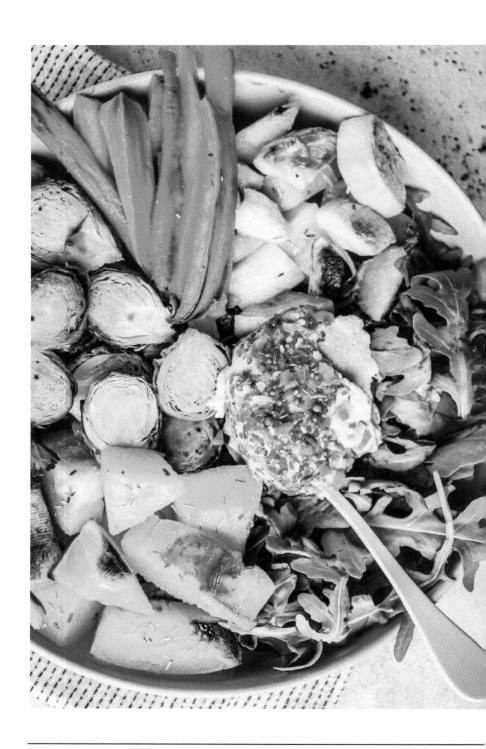

Grilled Kale Beets and Carrots

Ingredients:
- 1 bunch of Kale
- 5 pcs. Beets
- 2 medium Carrots, cut lengthwise and cut in half
- 4 large Tomatoes, sliced thick
- 1 large red onion, cut into 1/2 inch thick rounds
- 1/3 cup Italian parsley or basil, finely chopped

Dressing Ingredients:

- 6 tbsp. extra virgin olive oil
- 1 tsp. onion powder
- Sea salt, to taste
- 3 tbsp. distilled white vinegar
- 1 tsp. Dijon mustard

Directions:
1. Combine all of the dressing ingredients thoroughly.
2. Preheat your grill to low heat and grease the grates.

3. Layer the vegetables grill for 12 minutes per side, until tender flipping once.
4. Brush with the marinade/ dressing ingredients

Grilled Turnip Greens Okra and Red Onion

Ingredients:
- 1 bunch of turnip greens
- 10 pcs. Okra
- 1 large red onion, cut into 1/2 inch thick rounds
- 1/3 cup Italian parsley or basil, finely chopped
- 10 Broccolini Florets
- 10 pcs. Brussel Sprouts

Dressing Ingredients:
- 6 tbsp. olive oil
- 1 tsp. garlic powder
- 1 tsp. onion powder
- Sea salt, to taste
- 3 tbsp. white wine vinegar
- 1 tsp. English mustard

Directions:
1. Combine all of the dressing ingredients thoroughly.
2. Preheat your grill to low heat and grease the grates.

3. Layer the vegetables grill for 12 minutes per side, until tender flipping once.
4. Brush with the marinade/ dressing ingredients

Notes

Lightning Source UK Ltd.
Milton Keynes UK
UKHW020747030621
384855UK00001B/142